GUIDE to OPHTHALMIC AND NEUROLOGIC STEM CELL TREATMENTS

The Stem Cell Ophthalmology Treatment Study (SCOTS) and the Neurologic Stem Cell Study (NEST)

Jeffrey N. Weiss, M.D.

Steven Levy, M.D.

© 2016, Jeffrey N. Weiss, M.D.

DEDICATION

To our families, for our patients.

PREFACE

"It is not the critic who counts; not the man who points out how the strong man stumbles, or where the doer of deeds could have done them better. The credit belongs to the man who is actually in the arena, whose face is marred by dust and sweat and blood; who strives valiantly; who errs, who comes short again and again, because there is no effort without error and shortcoming; but who does actually strive to do the deeds; who knows great enthusiasms, the great devotions; who spends himself in a worthy cause; who at the best knows in the end the triumph of high achievement, and who at the worst, if he fails, at least fails while daring greatly, so that his place shall never be with those cold and timid souls who neither know victory nor defeat."

Theodore Roosevelt

"Two things are infinite: the universe and human stupidity; and I'm not sure about the universe."

Albert Einstein

"You are not entitled to your opinion. You are entitled to your *informed* opinion. No one is entitled to be ignorant."

Harlan Ellison

Chapter 1

What is Retinal and Optic Nerve Stem Cell Surgery?

There are many retinal and optic nerve conditions presently considered "untreatable." These conditions cause permanent visual loss, and natural history studies over the last 40 years have confirmed that there will not be a spontaneous improvement in vision. There are no treatments, and in many cases, none on the horizon.

Stem cells were discovered in 1981. Research, in animals, and now in humans, have demonstrated that the administration of bone-marrow derived stem cells (BMSC) can produce an improvement in vision in otherwise untreatable ophthalmic conditions.

In 2010, physicians in Dusseldorf, Germany were performing retrobulbar injections of BMSC to treat age-related macular degeneration (AMD) with good results. Dr. Weiss performed the first subretinal placement of BMSC on 2 American patients in Germany that same year. One of the patients regained the ability to read a large-print book (YouTube – retinal stem cell surgery).

Physicians in Tijuana, Mexico, were using intravitreal injections of adipose-derived stem cells (ADSC) to treat AMD with good results. However, Dr. Weiss examined a patient treated with ADSC that had developed proliferative vitreoretinopathy with a total retinal detachment, after receiving a subsequent intravitreal injection of Avastin for AMD. The pathology report of the vitreous specimen demonstrated adipose tissue. He has also heard of other complications in patients who received ADSC for ophthalmic conditions.

FDA regulations technically do not allow the use of ADSC for medical treatments outside of their approval. The FDA has ruled that the processing of the adipose tissue to isolate the stem cells is more than the "minimal manipulation" allowed by their regulations.

FDA regulations did allow the use of BMSC without their approval, although a recent change in their regulations only provides for "homologous use." This is a gray area as the bone marrow provides cells to all the organs in the body so technically the isolation of BMSC is in keeping with homologous use.

There is now extensive evidence the BMSC can regenerate non-hematopoietic tissues, including neural cells. Unlike embryonic stem cells, the use of BMSC avoids ethical issues.

The Stem Cell Ophthalmology Treatment Study (SCOTS) is an Institutional Board Approved Study registered with NIH. ClinicalTrials.gov Identifier: NCT01920867.

ClinicalTrials.gov

A service of the U.S. National Institutes of Health

Stem Cell Ophthalmology Treatment Study (SCOTS)

This study is currently recruiting participants. (see Contacts and Locations)
Verified January 2016 by Retina Associates of South Florida

Sponsor:

Retina Associates of South Florida

Collaborator:

MD Stem Cells

Information provided by (Responsible Party):

Retina Associates of South Florida

ClinicalTrials.gov Identifier:

NCT01920867

First received: August 8, 2013
Last updated: January 30, 2016
Last verified: January 2016

 Purpose

This study will evaluate the use of autologous bone marrow derived stem cells (BMSC) for the treatment of retinal and optic nerve damage or disease.

Condition
Retinal Disease   Procedure: RB (Retrobulbar)
Procedure: ST (Subtenon)
Procedure: IV (Intravenous)
Procedure: IVIT (Intravitreal)
Procedure: IO (Intraocular)
Macular Degeneration
Hereditary Retinal Dystrophy
Optic Nerve Disease
Glaucoma

Study Type:	Interventional
Study Design:	Allocation: Non-Randomized
	Endpoint Classification: Efficacy Study
	Intervention Model: Parallel Assignment
	Masking: Open Label
	Primary Purpose: Treatment
Official Title:	Bone Marrow Derived Stem Cell Ophthalmology Treatment Study

NLM links

Resource links provided by NLM:

ghr links
Genetics Home Reference related topics: age-related macular degeneration cone-rod dystrophy early-onset glaucoma neuromyelitis optica retinitis pigmentosa
medline links
MedlinePlus related topics: Macular Degeneration Neurologic Diseases Retinal Disorders
ORD links
Genetic and Rare Diseases Information Center resources: Neuromyelitis Optica Neuromyelitis Optica Spectrum Disorder Retinitis Pigmentosa Cone-rod Dystrophy Cone-rod Dystrophy 2 Stargardt Disease Optic Neuropathy, Anterior Ischemic Cone Dystrophy
U.S. FDA Resources

Further study details as provided by Retina Associates of South Florida:

primary outcomes
Primary Outcome Measures:

- Visual acuity [Time Frame: 1 day to 12 months] [Designated as safety issue: No]Best corrected visual acuity will be measured with Snellen Eye Chart and the ETDRS (Early Treatment Diabetic Retinopathy Study)Eye Chart when available at each post- procedure visit. Intervals at minimum will be first post- procedure day,then 3 months, 6 months and 12 months post-procedure day. Recommended visit 1 month post -procedure day.

secondary outcomes
Secondary Outcome Measures:

- Visual fields [Time Frame: 1 day to 12 months] [Designated as safety issue: No]Visual fields will be evaluated with automated perimetry during post- procedure visits as needed and specifically at 6 months and 12 months.

Estimated Enrollment:	300
Study Start Date:	August 2013
Estimated Study Completion Date:	August 2017
Estimated Primary Completion Date:	August 2016 (Final data collection date for primary outcome measure)

arms and groups table

Arms	Assigned Interventions
Active Comparator: RB, ST, IV Injections of BMSC retrobulbar (RB), subtenon (ST) and intravenous (IV)	Procedure: RB (Retrobulbar) Retrobulbar injection of Bone Marrow Derived Stem Cells (BMSC) Other Name: Retrobulbar injection of stem cells Procedure: ST (Subtenon) Subtenon injection of Bone Marrow Derived Stem Cells (BMSC) Other Name: Subtenon injection of stem cells Procedure: IV (Intravenous) Intravenous injection of Bone Marrow Derived Stem Cells (BMSC) Other Name: Intravenous injection of stem cells
Active Comparator: RB, ST, IV, IVIT Injections of BMSC retrobulbar, subtenon, intravenous and intravitreal (IVIT)	Procedure: RB (Retrobulbar) Retrobulbar injection of Bone Marrow Derived Stem Cells (BMSC) Other Name: Retrobulbar injection of stem cells Procedure: ST (Subtenon) Subtenon injection of Bone Marrow Derived Stem Cells (BMSC) Other Name: Subtenon injection of stem cells Procedure: IV (Intravenous) Intravenous injection of Bone Marrow Derived Stem Cells (BMSC)

	Other Name: Intravenous injection of stem cells Procedure: IVIT (Intravitreal) Intravitreal injection of Bone Marrow Derived Stem Cells (BMSC) Other Name: Intravitreal injection of stem cells
Active Comparator: RB, ST, IV, IO Injection of BMSC retrobulbar, subtenon, intravenous and intraocular (IO) with vitrectomy	Procedure: RB (Retrobulbar) Retrobulbar injection of Bone Marrow Derived Stem Cells (BMSC) Other Name: Retrobulbar injection of stem cells Procedure: ST (Subtenon) Subtenon injection of Bone Marrow Derived Stem Cells (BMSC) Other Name: Subtenon injection of stem cells Procedure: IV (Intravenous) Intravenous injection of Bone Marrow Derived Stem Cells (BMSC) Other Name: Intravenous injection of stem cells Procedure: IO (Intraocular) Intraocular injection of Bone Marrow Derived Stem Cells (BMSC) with vitrectomy prior to intraocular injection. For example, may include larger amount of stem cells in the intravitreal cavity, intraneuronal injections or subretinal injections of stem cells. Other Name: Intraocular injection of stem cells with vitrectomy

Detailed Description:

Eyes with loss of vision from retinal or optic nerve conditions generally considered irreversible will be treated with a combination of injections of autologous bone marrow derived stem cells isolated from the bone marrow using standard medical and surgical practices. Retinal conditions may include degenerative, ischemic or physical damage (examples may include macular degeneration, hereditary retinal dystrophies such as retinitis pigmentosa, stargardt, non-perfusion retinopathies, post retinal detachment. Optic Nerve conditions may include degenerative, ischemic or physical damage (examples may include optic nerve damage from glaucoma, compression, ischemic optic neuropathy, optic atrophy). Injections may include retrobulbar, subtenon, intravitreal, intraocular, subretinal and intravenous. Patients will be followed for 12 months with serial comprehensive eye examinations including relevant imaging and diagnostic ophthalmic testing.

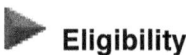 **Eligibility**

Ages Eligible for Study:	18 Years and older (Adult, Senior)
Genders Eligible for Study:	Both
Accepts Healthy Volunteers:	No

Criteria

Inclusion Criteria:

- Have objective, documented damage to the retina or optic nerve unlikely to improve OR
- Have objective, documented damage to the retina or optic nerve that is progressive
- AND have less than or equal to 20/40 best corrected central visual acuity in one or both eyes AND/OR an abnormal visual field in one or both eyes.

- Be at least 3 months post-surgical treatment intended to treat any ophthalmologic disease and stable.
- If under current medical therapy (pharmacologic treatment) for a retinal or optic nerve disease be considered stable on that treatment and unlikely to have visual function improvement (for example, glaucoma with intraocular pressure stable on topical medications but visual field damage).
- Have the potential for improvement with BMSC treatment and be at minimal risk of any potential harm from the procedure.
- Be over the age of 18
- Be medically stable and able to be medically cleared by their primary care physician or a licensed primary care practitioner for the procedure. Medical clearance means that in the estimation of the primary care practitioner, the patient can reasonably be expected to undergo the procedure without significant medical risk to health.

Exclusion Criteria:

- Patients who are not capable of an adequate ophthalmologic examination or evaluation to document the pathology.
- Patients who are not capable or not willing to undergo follow up eye exams with the principle investigator or their ophthalmologist or optometrist as outlined in the protocol.
- Patients who are not capable of providing informed consent.
- Patients who may be at significant risk to general health or to the eyes and visual function should they undergo the procedure.

Contacts and Locations

Choosing to participate in a study is an important personal decision. Talk with your doctor and family members or friends about deciding to join a study. To learn more about this study, you or your doctor may contact the study research staff using the Contacts provided below. For general information, see Learn About Clinical Studies.

Please refer to this study by its ClinicalTrials.gov identifier: NCT01920867

Contacts

Contact: Steven Levy, MD   203-423-9494   stevenlevy@mdstemcells.com

Locations

United States, Florida

Retina Associates of South Florida   **Recruiting**
Margate, Florida, United States, 33063
Contact: Steven Levy, MD   203-423-9494   stevenlevy@mdstemcells.com
Principal Investigator: Jeffrey Weiss, MD
Sub-Investigator: Steven Levy, MD

United Arab Emirates

Al Zahra Hospital   **Recruiting**
Dubai, United Arab Emirates
Contact: Steven Levy, MD   (001)203-423-9494   stevenlevy@mdstemcells.com

Sponsors and Collaborators

Retina Associates of South Florida
MD Stem Cells

Investigators

Principal Investigator:	Jeffrey Weiss, MD	Retina Associates of South Florida
Study Director:	Steven Levy, MD	MD Stem Cells

 More Information

Additional Information:

The Role of Patient Funded Clinical Research in Advancing Medical Care

Publications:

Weiss JN, Levy S, Malkin A. Stem Cell Ophthalmology Treatment Study (SCOTS) for retinal and optic nerve diseases: a preliminary report. Neural Regen Res. 2015 Jun;10(6):982-8. doi: 10.4103/1673-5374.158365.

Weiss JN, Levy S, Benes SC. Stem Cell Ophthalmology Treatment Study (SCOTS) for retinal and optic nerve diseases: a case report of improvement in relapsing auto-immune optic neuropathy. Neural Regen Res. 2015 Sep;10(9):1507-15. doi: 10.4103/1673-5374.165525.

Available Study Data/Document Available Study Data/Document

Responsible Party:	Retina Associates of South Florida
ClinicalTrials.gov Identifier:	NCT01920867 History of Changes
Other Study ID Numbers:	ICMS-2013-0019.
Study First Received:	August 8, 2013
Last Updated:	January 30, 2016
Health Authority:	United States: Institutional Review Board United States: Federal Government United States: Data and Safety Monitoring Board

keywords

Keywords provided by Retina Associates of South Florida:

Stem Cells
Dry Macular Degeneration
Wet Macular Degeneration
Retinal Atrophy
Retinal Dystrophy
Hereditary Retinal Dystrophy
Retinitis Pigmentosa
Stargardt's Disease
Cone Dystrophy
Cone Rod Dystrophy
Maculopathy
Optic Nerve Disease
Optic Nerve Atrophy
Optic Atrophy
Ischemic Optic Neuropathy
Wet Macular Degeneration
Retinal Atrophy
Retinal Dystrophy
Hereditary Retinal Dystrophy
Retinitis Pigmentosa
Stargardt Disease

Cone Dystrophy
Cone Rod Dystrophy
Maculopathy
Optic Nerve Disease
Optic Nerve Atrophy
Optic Atrophy
Ischemic Optic
Bone Marrow Derived Stem Cells
BMSC
BMC (Bone Marrow Cell)
Mesenchymal Stem Cells
MSC
Eye Disease
Eye Stem Cells
Ophthalmology
Ophthalmic Disease
Retina
Retinal Disease
Macular Degeneration
Age Related Macular Degeneration
Myopic Macular Degeneration

mesh terms
Additional relevant MeSH terms:

Glaucoma
Ocular Hypertension
Eye Diseases
Retinal Degeneration
Cranial Nerve Dis
Macular Degeneration
Retinal Diseases
Retinal Dystrophies
Nervous System Diseases

Institutional Review Board approval in the U.S. is limited to those patient 18 years of age and older. We are able to treat patients younger than 18 years of age at Al Zahra Hospital in Dubai. This is a modern, state of the art hospital with excellent support services. The hospital is approved by the U.S. Joint Commission on Accreditation.

PROCEDURE

Patients first contact the SCOTS Study Director, Dr. Steven Levy, the President of MD Stem Cells. Dr. Levy provides information and manages the logistics and data for the study. Patient ophthalmic records are sent to Dr. Levy at stevenlevy@mdstemcells.com.

Dr. Levy forwards the records to Dr. Jeffrey Weiss, the Principal Investigator of SCOTS and a practicing retinal specialist in Margate, Florida, for review. Dr. Weiss independently determines patient eligibility. He will also select the best procedure for the patient. Dr. Weiss performs all ophthalmic surgeries.

The surgery is usually performed using general anesthesia, and takes less than 1 hour. A state-of-the-art outpatient surgery center is used for all procedures. An orthopedic surgeon performs the bone marrow aspiration and the bone marrow fraction (BMF), which consists of the stem cells and multiple growth factors, is isolated using our protocol in an FDA approved Class 2 device.

In SCOTS, there is the choice of 3 ophthalmic procedures:

Arm 1 consists of a retrobulbar and a subtenons injection of the BMF. A retrobulbar injection is the placement of cells behind the eye. A subtenons injection is the placement of cells between the sclera, or white part of the eye, and the overlying transparent tissue.

Arm 2 consists of the Arm 1 procedures and an intravitreal injection. An intravitreal injection is injecting the cells into the eye.

Arm 3 is a vitrectomy and subtenons injection. A vitrectomy is a surgical procedure that is used to remove the vitreous body from inside the eye. The vitreous material is replaced with a saline solution. The vitrectomy allows the surgeon access to directly inject cells into the optic nerve or under the retina.

The procedures are tailored for the individual patient. The patient may have Arm 1 or 2 in one or both eyes, but Arm 3 is reserved for one eye, and for the eye with the worst visual acuity. As of this date we have performed the SCOTS surgery on more than 400 patients, and more than 750 eyes.

Experience has shown that the direct placement of the BMF under the retina may be beneficial for certain diseases that affect the macula - the center portion of the retina. However for many retinal diseases including different macular diseases, improvements in vision have been seen in patients receiving Arm 1 or 2 injections alone.

Similarly, direct injection of the optic nerve may be provided in specific cases as the cells seem to remain over time. However the optic nerve actually forms from the nerve fiber layer, a portion of the retina - therefore Arm 1 or 2 injections alone are sufficient to see improvements in many cases.

There have been no complications in patients undergoing Arm 1 or 2. In the first 100 Arm 3 cases there were 3 retinal detachments where a commercially available needle was used to inject the cells. All 3 cases were successfully repaired. As a result of this experience, Dr. Weiss developed his own subretinal needles and since utilizing these needles there have been no retinal detachments.

Experience has shown that eyes in each of the categories, improve. The choice of which Arm of the procedure the patient receives is based on the ophthalmic history and the clinical examination.

In Arm 3 for retinal cases, Dr. Weiss performs a vitrectomy and then using a needle of his design, places the BMF in the area of atrophic retina.

In the Arm 3 optic nerve cases, following the vitrectomy, there is a direct injection of the BMF cells into the optic nerve. If the visual acuity is sufficient to perform a visual field test, Dr. Weiss uses the field to guide the injection into atrophic nerve.

In either Arm 1 or 2, the eye is not patched. The eye undergoing Arm 3 is patched for 24 hours.

The patients are instructed to not rub their eyes, to avoid heavy lifting and straining, and in the Arm 2 and 3 eyes, to keep their "head above their heart" and sleep on 2 pillows until the "floaters" are gone.

It is important to note that the BMF is red in color. Our cell separation protocol has been developed over 4 years and been modified and improved multiple times in order to minimize the presence of red blood cells.

Typically Arm 1 and Arm 2 patients will postoperatively exhibit inferior orbital discoloration, and subconjunctival redness. This is the color of the BMF, it is not hemorrhage. Arm 2 patients will look like there is a "vitreous hemorrhage," but it is not hemorrhage, but the BMF.

The intravitreal BMF generally is clumped inferiorly, but in a vitrectomized eye, or an eye that has experienced a posterior vitreous detachment with a very "liquidy" vitreous, the cells will dissipate giving the impression of a vitreous hemorrhage. This may also be seen in Arm 3 eyes treated for a retinal condition in that some of the BMF may remain in the vitreous cavity. In those Arm 3 eyes that underwent direct injection of the BMF into the optic disc, though there may not be any BMF in the vitreous cavity at the conclusion of surgery, some of the BMF material may be visible overlying the optic disc on the first postoperative day.

Knowing what to expect is important. We have had one case in which the patient returned home after SCOTS treatment, her ophthalmologist saw a "vitreous hemorrhage" and he immediately performed a vitrectomy to remove the BMF that we placed!

Arm 1 and Arm 2 patients report that their eyes feel "scratchy". The discomfort is generally gone by the first postoperative day. Arm 3 eyes are patched until the first postoperative day, and then the patient may feel a foreign body sensation for a few days. All patients report either slight, or no hip discomfort after surgery.

The patients are instructed to refrain from straining activities, such as heavy lifting and to keep their head "above their heart" for one month after surgery. The Arm 3 patients are advised to wear glasses or a metal shield when they sleep, for one month after surgery.

Data is collected at 1, 3, 6 and 12 months postoperatively. The post surgical examinations are generally performed by the patient's local eye doctor. The information we request is: visual acuity, eye pressure, anterior and posterior segment examinations, fundus photography, Optical Coherence Tomography (OCT) and visual fields.

The periorbital and subconjunctival redness, and the intravitreal BMF material generally resolve with one month. We have seen improvements in visual acuity on the first postoperative day although generally improvement is noted from 4 to 6 months after the procedure. We have had one patient who suddenly experienced visual improvement 8 months after surgery. If patients wish to repeat the procedure they should wait one year in order to be in compliance with the SCOTS protocol. .

The first patient to undergo the SCOTS procedure has incrementally experienced improvements in his vision each year after repeating the procedure. He has now undergone the SCOTS procedure 4 times. During the 4 years he improved from sitting in a chair in his mother's house, to meeting a girl, purchasing a home, resume the practice of law (by enlarging the print on a computer) and marrying.

An increasing number of patient who have previously improved, have asked to return to repeat the surgery in the hope of achieving further visual gains.

Since more than 95% of our patients come to us from out of state or out of the country, the postoperative data is collected by a physician unrelated to us or SCOTS. In some cases the physician has been hostile to the patient concerning their involvement in SCOTS and that makes communications difficult.

When the patient is to return home after surgery, they are given a chart detailing what testing is required at the 1, 3, 6 and 12 month postoperative visits. In addition, they are given copies of the patient's preoperative visit (Monday) and the last postoperative visit (Friday).

In the past we told the patient to ask the physician to send us the postoperative data. In order to increase the receipt of this important information, we now instruct the patients to ask for a copy of their records at the time of their examination and send them to us. There has been an exponential increase in the number of records we now receive.

Helping patients who have never been helped before makes all the hard work extremely worthwhile.

Chapter 2

What is the Neurology Stem Cell Treatment Study? (NEST)

We had noticed improvements in patients treated in SCOTS who also had neurologic conditions. One patient had lost the ability to smell and had persistent ringing in his ears since experiencing head trauma more than 20 years earlier. Two days after he underwent the surgery, the ringing in his ears stopped and his sense of smell returned. One patient no longer needed to use a walker. Another was able to speak again after a stroke. These observations formed the basis for the NEST study, the Neurology Stem Cell Treatment Study.

We recently submitted the NEST protocol to the IRB and it was approved. The study is registered with the NIH and appears on its website, ClinicalTrials.gov Identifier NCT0279052, as was done with SCOTS.

In NEST, our protocol treats patients with chronic Traumatic Brain Injury, Parkinson's Disease, Multiple Sclerosis and Diabetic Neuropathy. The procedure consists of the bone marrow aspiration under anesthesia and the separation of the stem cells, as in SCOTS.

In NEST, the patient receives the bone marrow aspirate material (BMF) and stem cells intravenously and intranasally via aerosol. The surgery is generally performed under monitored anesthesia. The procedure takes approximately 30 minutes and is performed at the same out-patient surgery center we use for SCOTS.

Data is collected by the patient's referring neurologist at the 1, 3, 6, and 12 month postoperative examinations.

ClinicalTrials.gov

A service of the U.S. National Institutes of Health

Neurologic Stem Cell Treatment Study (NEST)

This study is currently recruiting participants. (see **Contacts and Locations**)

Verified June 2016 by Retina Associates of South Florida

Sponsor:

Retina Associates of South Florida

Collaborator:

MD **Stem Cells**
Information provided by (Responsible Party):
Retina Associates of South Florida

ClinicalTrials.gov Identifier:

NCT02795052
First received: June 6, 2016
Last updated: June 19, 2016
Last verified: June 2016

▶ Purpose

This is a human clinical **study** involving the isolation of autologous bone marrow derived **stem cells** (BMSC) and transfer to the vascular system and/ or cribriform plate area in order to determine if such a treatment will provide a statistically significant improvement in neurologic function for patients with certain neurologic conditions.

Condition
Neurologic Disorders
Procedure: Intravenous
BMSC
Procedure: Intranasal
BMSC
Nervous System Diseases
Neurodegenerative Diseases
Neurological Disorders

Study Type: Interventional
Study Design: Allocation: Non-Randomized
Endpoint Classification: Efficacy **Study**
Intervention Model: Parallel Assignment
Masking: Open Label
Primary Purpose: Treatment
Official Title: Neurologic Bone Marrow Derived **Stem Cell** Treatment **Study**

NLM links
Resource links provided by NLM:

medline links
MedlinePlus related topics: Neurologic Diseases
U.S. FDA Resources

Further study details as provided by Retina Associates of South Florida:

primary outcomes
Primary Outcome Measures:

- Activities of Daily Living (ADL) [Time Frame: 3 to 12 months] [Designated as safety issue: No]Activities of Daily Living (ADL) will be assessed at 3,6 and 12 months following the procedure

Secondary Outcome Measures:

- Neurologic Functioning [Time Frame: 3 to 12 months]
  [Designated as safety issue: No]Deficits of neurologic function identified by the patient as impaired prior to treatment will be assessed. As examples, neurologic functions may include speech, balance, hearing, gait, strength, pain, paresthesias, etc.

Estimated Enrollment:	300
Study Start Date:	June 2016
Estimated Study Completion Date:	June 2021
Estimated Primary Completion Date:	June 2020 (Final data collection date for primary outcome measure)

arms and groups table

Arms
Active Comparator: Arm 1 - Intravenous BMSC Intervention- Autologous bone marrow aspiration and separation of Bone Marrow Derived **Stem Cell** (BMSC) fraction then provided intravenously.
Active Comparator: Arm 2- Intravenous and Intranasal BMSC Intervention- Autologous bone marrow aspiration and separation of Bone Marrow Derived **Stem Cell** (BMSC) fraction then provided intravenously and intranasally.

Detailed Description:

Various clinical studies have registered with the National Institutes of Health (NIH) to study neurologic diseases and damage. There have also been a number of journal reports of the benefits of treatment with BMSC for diseases and damage to nervous tissue. The investigators hope to add to the volume of literature regarding the use of BMSC in those neurologic diseases and conditions identified as likely to respond to this treatment.

Intravenous administration of BMSC is a well-established approach to neurologic disease and injury with much support for its effectiveness in the pre-clinical and clinical literature. BMSC and the associated bone marrow fraction are posited to have a number of different mechanisms by which they may potentially improve neurologic function. In regards to their ability to penetrate the blood-brain barrier, within the diencephalon there are specific circumventricular organs which lie in the wall of the third ventricle. These are noteworthy for lacking a tight blood-brain barrier so that the brain may coordinate endocrine and nervous systems functions including blood pressure, fluid balance, hunger and thirst. Entry of BMSC into the brain via intravenous administration through these circumventricular organs has been documented by researchers.

In addition to the use of intravenous BMSC, the NEST Study provides a treatment arm using application of BMSC to the cribriform plate in the upper nasal passages as a means of introducing BMSC to the Central Nervous System (CNS). The cribriform plate is an area of the ethmoid bone at the superior portion of the nasal cavity where the primary olfactory nerves enter the CNS. Within the cribriform plate there are approximately 40 tiny openings through which the axons of the primary olfactory sensory neurons pass into the CNS and synapse with the secondary neurons forming the olfactory bulb that continues as the olfactory nerve. There is significant documentation in the literature that intranasal delivery follows the pathways of both the olfactory and trigeminal nerves, facilitating entry into the parenchyma and cerebral spinal fluid (CSF) for effects on the CNS.

▶ Eligibility

Ages Eligible for Study:	18 Years and older (Adult, Senior)
Genders Eligible for Study:	Both

Accepts Healthy Volunteers: No

Criteria

Inclusion Criteria:

- Have documented functional damage to the central or peripheral nervous system unlikely to improve with present standard of care.
- Be at least 6 months post-onset of the disease.
- If under current medical therapy (pharmacologic or surgical treatment) for the condition be considered stable on that treatment and unlikely to have reversal of the associated neurologic functional damage as a result of the ongoing pharmacologic or surgical treatment.
- In the estimation of Dr. Weiss and the neurologists have the potential for improvement with BMSC treatment and be at minimal risk of any potential harm from the procedure.
- Be over the age of 18 and capable of providing informed consent.
- Be medically stable and able to be medically cleared by their primary care physician or a licensed primary care practitioner for the procedure. Medical clearance means that in the estimation of the primary care practitioner, the patient can reasonably be expected to undergo the procedure without significant medical risk to health.

Exclusion Criteria:

- All patients must be capable of an adequate neurologic examination and evaluation to document the pathology. This will include the ability to cooperate with the exam.
- Patients must be capable and willing to undergo follow up neurologic exams with the sub-investigators or their own neurologists as outlined in the protocol.
- Patients must be capable of providing informed consent.
- In the estimation of Dr. Weiss the BMSC collection and treatment will not present a significant risk of harm to the patient's general health or to their neurologic function. .

- Patients who are not medically stable or who may be at significant risk to their health undergoing the procedure will not be eligible.
- Women of childbearing age must not be pregnant at the time of treatment and should refrain from becoming pregnant for 3 months post treatment.

▶ Contacts and Locations

Choosing to participate in a study is an important personal decision. Talk with your doctor and family members or friends about deciding to join a study. To learn more about this study, you or your doctor may contact the study research staff using the Contacts provided below. For general information, see Learn About Clinical Studies.

Please refer to this study by its ClinicalTrials.gov identifier: NCT02795052

Contacts

Contact: Steven Levy, MD   203-423-9494   stevenlevy@mdstemcells.com

Locations

United States, Florida

Retina Associates of South Florida   **Recruiting**
Margate, Florida, United States, 33063
Contact: Steven Levy, MD   203-423-9494   stevenlevy@mdstemcells.com

United Arab Emirates

Al Zahra Hospital   **Recruiting**
Dubai, United Arab Emirates
Contact: Steven Levy, MD   203-423-9494   stevenlevy@mdstemcells.com

Sponsors and Collaborators

Retina Associates of South Florida

MD **Stem Cells**

Investigators

Study Director:	Steven Levy, MD	MD **Stem Cells**
Principal Investigator:	Jeffrey Weiss, MD	Retina Associates of South Florida

▶ More Information

Publications:

Chapman CD, Frey WH 2nd, Craft S, Danielyan L, Hallschmid M, Schiöth HB, Benedict C. Intranasal treatment of central nervous system dysfunction in humans. Pharm Res. 2013 Oct;30(10):2475-84. doi: 10.1007/s11095-012-0915-1. Epub 2012 Nov 8. Review.

Jiang Y, Zhu J, Xu G, Liu X. Intranasal delivery of stem cells to the brain. Expert Opin Drug Deliv. 2011 May;8(5):623-32. doi: 10.1517/17425247.2011.566267. Epub 2011 Mar 19. Review.

Bhasin A, Srivastava M, Bhatia R, Mohanty S, Kumaran S, Bose S. Autologous intravenous mononuclear stem cell therapy in chronic ischemic stroke. J Stem Cells Regen Med. 2012 Nov 26;8(3):181-9. eCollection 2012.

Teixeira FG, Carvalho MM, Sousa N, Salgado AJ. Mesenchymal stem cells secretome: a new paradigm for central nervous system regeneration? Cell Mol Life Sci. 2013 Oct;70(20):3871-82. doi: 10.1007/s00018-013-1290-8. Epub 2013 Mar 1. Review.

Lescaudron L, Naveilhan P, Neveu I. The use of stem cells in regenerative medicine for Parkinson's and Huntington's Diseases. Curr Med Chem. 2012;19(35):6018-35. Review.

Laroni A, de Rosbo NK, Uccelli A. Mesenchymal stem cells for the treatment of neurological diseases: Immunoregulation beyond neuroprotection. Immunol Lett. 2015 Dec;168(2):183-90. doi: 10.1016/j.imlet.2015.08.007. Epub 2015 Aug 18.

Anbari F, Khalili MA, Bahrami AR, Khoradmehr A, Sadeghian F, Fesahat F, Nabi A. Intravenous transplantation of bone marrow mesenchymal stem cells promotes neural regeneration after traumatic brain injury. Neural Regen Res. 2014 May 1;9(9):919-23. doi: 10.4103/1673-5374.133133.

Available Study Data/Document Available Study Data/Document

Responsible Party:	Retina Associates of South Florida
ClinicalTrials.gov Identifier:	NCT02795052 History of Changes
Other Study ID Numbers:	MDSC-**NEST**
Study First Received:	June 6, 2016
Last Updated:	June 19, 2016
Health Authority:	United States: Institutional Review Board United States: Data and Safety Monitoring Board

Keywords provided by Retina Associates of South Florida:

Neurologic Disease
Cerebral Vascular Accident
Stroke
Traumatic Brain Injury
Multiple Sclerosis
Parkinson's Disease
Neuropathy

Neurodegeneration
Diabetic Neuropathy
Cerebral Ischemia

Disease
Nervous System Diseases
Neurodegenerative Diseases
Pathologic Processes

CONCLUSION

The decision to participate in a new treatment requires careful consideration. Discuss this information with your family, friends, and your physician. We hope the information presented in this book will help you in making a decision regarding participation. If you have questions, or require additional information, please contact Dr. Steven Levy at: stevenlevy@mdstemcells.com.

Addendum 1

Frequently Asked Questions about the Stem Cell Ophthalmology Treatment Study (SCOTS)

1. Why do you charge patients for an "experimental" procedure?

All human endeavors, including clinical research, must be paid for. When patients think of clinical studies, they usually think of pharmaceutical companies doing research to obtain FDA approval for their drug. Pharmaceutical companies have a patent on a drug and investments are made into research and clinical studies in hopes of obtaining FDA approval, recouping investments and earning profits by charging patients who use the drug. SCOTS and NEST are not patented processes and there is no one investing in these procedures. In order to provide this care and advance regenerative medicine, we must charge the patients for the procedures.

We have never had a complaint from any patient participating in these studies about our charges for the procedure. They understand the reasons.

Stem cells were discovered in 1981. SCOTS began in 2012. As of this date there is not another study like it in the world. If SCOTS did not exist, the almost 400 patients we have treated would still not have been treated.

There is no proprietary drug at the end of the study. In fact, with the exception of the needles Dr. Weiss developed for the retinal surgery, nothing is proprietary. There is no patent protection. A pharmaceutical company cannot make a billion dollars profit, like they do with erectile dysfunction drugs. So who is to pay for it? The government?

Government funding is given to research prominent life threatening conditions such as cancer and HIV/AIDS, and is awarded to Universities and not to physicians in private practice. A private foundation? They support their own causes, have limited resources and are guided by academics that tend to support their own, other academics. A private doctor working in his own office will not receive a grant.

The fact that Dr. Weiss taught at Harvard Medical School, was Chief of Retinal Surgery at the Joslin Diabetes Center in Boston, was tenured, ran a research laboratory that received government and private grants, taught fellows to be retinal specialists, was a Visiting Scientist at M.I.T. is completely discounted. They don't remove your brain or your desire to do research when you leave academics.

One reason Dr. Weiss left the academic institution was because the research there was smothered by bureaucracy and overhead costs. Dr. Weiss is able to perform better and more efficient research in an environment he controls, not one controlled by people without any sense of urgency to whom one research project is the same as any other.

Unlike a drug company study in which the treatment is free, our patients are much better informed; after all, it is their own money they are spending. Anyone has the right to spend money on anything they choose. One can purchase liquor, tobacco, firearms, a house or car that they cannot safely afford without any interference. Yet, physicians who have done nothing to help these patients, who tell them to return for another visit in 6 months and charge them for the examination, only to yet again tell them that there is nothing they can do, criticize us for charging patients.

How moral is it to hold yourself out as an expert, yet be unaware of a study, listed on ClinicalTrials.gov, the NIH website, that might help the patient you are charging? And what do they offer in return? Nothing. We find it distressing that physicians who are able to see, make pronouncements about what blind patients should do, when you know that if they became blind, they would be contacting us for inclusion in our study.

2. Why are you killing babies?

The answer – we are not. This is the second most common question we hear. This work has nothing to do with embryonic or fetal stem cells. These are the patient's own stem cells - termed autologous. The bone marrow stem cells are taken from the patient during the surgical procedure. Approximately 5 – 10% of the patients in SCOTS have initially been refused postoperative examinations by their own eye doctors because the doctors have misunderstood the source of the stem cells.

3. Why haven't you published your results in the mainstream ophthalmic journals?

We have tried. The mainstream ophthalmic journals have returned our papers without comment, or made comments we felt were inappropriate. Publishing is not free, in fact, each paper may cost us several thousand dollars to be published. That is why we are publishing in a stem cell journal that is on-line, is peer reviewed, and is listed on the U.S. government Library of Medicine website, PubMed.gov. We have published 3 articles, have another article in review, and are writing more articles. The people criticizing us have never read out articles, nor our protocol. An opinion not based upon fact is a prejudice.

Not publishing in a mainstream journal doesn't mean the work isn't good. The reviewers are anonymous, but the authors are not. Prior studies have shown that there is bias in selecting papers for publication. Whether the authors are at a large institution, associated with the government, or at a drug company, has been found to impact the acceptance of an article. If the research is excellent, but the paper is not as excellent, the article may not be published. The disconnect between the research and its publication prevents the dissemination of knowledge.

In Dr. Weiss's career as an ophthalmologist and a researcher, he has had articles rejected because they didn't include photos; the photos were then included and then the article was rejected because it contained photos. Articles he submitted were held by the journal for many months longer than they should have been, only to find that another article on a similar topic was published; in one case, containing paragraphs lifted from the article Dr. Weiss had written. Letters to the Editor have been published taking credit for, or ridiculing Dr. Weiss's work, but the Editor of the journal refused to allow him to respond.

One of the more ridiculous responses was in regard to the article written by Dr. Weiss concerning the use of hyperbaric oxygen to treat retinal arterial occlusions, a condition causing the loss of vision or even blindness. The article was accepted pending revision. Dr. Weiss made the required revisions and then the article was rejected because it was not relevant to the eye. Treating retinal artery occlusions that cause the loss of vision with good results was not relevant?

If publishing is the "gold standard" then it should be transparent.

4. Why is the your work considered experimental?

The definition of experimental is the use of untested ideas or techniques that are not yet established or finalized. This was true of the first cases of each of the 47 different conditions, and mixed conditions, we have treated. The fact that approximately 60% of the patients have experienced visual improvement have established the idea and technique. People often criticize what they don't understand.

To quote Max Planck, the great German physicist,
"A new scientific truth does not triumph by convincing its opponents and making them see the light, but rather because its opponents eventually die, and a new generation grows up that is familiar with it." The history of medicine is replete with many examples of pioneers being attacked and ridiculed. The following

generation of physicians, with no preconceived notions or axes to grind, accept the work.

5. Why haven't you performed animal studies.

Thousands of animal studies have been performed and the data is available on PubMed, the National Library of Medicine website. Rather then reinventing the wheel, science is advanced by building on the work of others, not by repeating it. On the basis of the animal studies, various centers around the world were performing clinical studies. Dr. Weiss visited these centers and learned from them. Only then was the SCOTS protocol written and submitted to the Institutional Review Board for approval.

6. When will insurance companies pay for the SCOTS procedure?

Insurance companies are profit-generating businesses. The less they pay out, the more profitable they are. Everything is experimental until there are many double blind control clinical studies, which they won't pay for, that proves the treatment works. Since there is little funding, and it takes a generation for a new controversial medical treatment to be accepted, insurance companies won't be paying for the SCOTS treatment for quite a while.

7. When will SCOTS end?

We were recently approved for an additional 500 patients. As long as patients are being helped, we don't expect SCOTS to end.

8. Why is the treatment so expensive?

There are many people involved in the study. The price includes payment for the anesthesiologist, the orthopedic surgeon, 2 ophthalmologists, the company that provides the stem cell separation equipment and all the disposable equipment, the surgery center and personnel, etc. We asked a University that was referring patients to SCOTS to determine what their charges would be for the same procedure and their charges would have been significantly higher than ours.

9. How do patients pay for the study?

Patients typically have their own resources or have help from family or friends. Sometimes they have raised funds through donation requests through work or their religious affiliations. Not uncommonly they have raised portions or even the entire amount through websites helping people to connect with donors such as www.gofundme.com. They have contacted local newspapers that have written stories about their blindness and SCOTS, which has assisted them in raising funds. Usually where there is a will, there is a way. Sadly, their requests to prominent eye organizations which sometimes collect millions of dollars in donations to support research involving their particular disease have typically not resulted in any direct help.

Addendum 2

The Role of Patient Funded Clinical Research in Advancing Medical Care

A clinical trial, also called an interventional trial, is a type of research where participants receive a specific intervention that is dictated by a study protocol. The intervention may be a surgical procedure, drug, device, or change to the participants behavior, such as a diet. Clinical trials may compare a new medical or surgical approach to no intervention. There are various sources that provide funding for clinical trials.

The National Institutes of Health (NIH)

The NIH is the largest biomedical funding source in the U.S. There has been a 20% inflation adjusted decline in the NIH budget over the last decade. Approximately 15 – 20 % of grant submissions receive funding and due to government budget sequestration, investigators receive only 90% of the approved funds. A 2007 U.S. government study found that university faculty members spend approximately 40% of their research time navigating bureaucracy.

A research grant is awarded to an individual at a university, but not to the same individual when he enters private practice, effectively removing an experienced researcher from government funding. NIH grants are typically for a 3 year period and end abruptly if not renewed. In addition, the researcher is unable to shift the funds to another project if the first project is not successful.

Best has demonstrated that disease advocacy has political outcomes, including direct benefits, distributive changes and systemic effects. She has shown that advocacy groups secure gains for their members (direct benefits), that the mobilized groups receive resources at the expense of the elite political influence (distributive changes) and that such groups can change the system of political decision making (systemic effects).

Pharmaceutical Companies

Pharmaceutical Companies are commercial enterprises organized to make money. Approximately 75% of clinical trials in medicine are company sponsored. Such funding may introduce bias, as the study design or interpretation is more likely to favor the drug under consideration with the ultimate goal, the attainment of FDA approval. This is understandable as the time to develop a successful drug is 10 to 15 years and the cost to achieve FDA approval has successively increased over the decades to approximately 1.2 billion dollars at the present time.

An orphan disease is defined as any disease affecting up to 200,000 individuals in the U.S. There are incentives offered to pharmaceutical companies through the Orphan Drug Act of 1983 to address the rare disease market. However orphan diseases with larger numbers of patients or those diseases for which there may be less price resistance regarding any successful treatment may draw development efforts in an unfair way.

Non-Profit Organizations

Like the NIH, non-profits use a panel of expert who decide the worthiness of a particular grant and determine the awarding of funding. As such, they suffer from the same problem as the NIH.

Thomas Kuhn has pointed out that breakthrough insights frequently stem from the intersection of disciplines, not from within the discipline. Grant reviewers are generally within the same discipline and can't recognize the new paradigm that may have come from the work of scientists in other fields. They remain committed to the old paradigm that has shaped their beliefs, which prompted Max Planck to say, "New scientific truth does not triumph by convincing its opponents and making them see the light, but rather because its opponents eventually die, and a new generation grows up that is familiar with it." Also like the NIH, nonprofit organizations award grants to institutions, not to individual researchers in private practice.

Private Funded Research

This includes a broad pool of donors with a wide range of passions that may speed progress by investing in bold ideas, gambles, and risky projects. Decisions may be made quickly, not encumbered by large bureaucracies. A sense of urgency can be respected.

Critics argue that gifts privatize research and steer resources towards areas of personal interest. Supporters argue that it is the personal choice of the funder whether money is spent on personal goods or personal research. Personally funded projects have a vested interest in solving the chosen problem and, unlike pharmaceutically funded research, are not subject to the profit motive or market forces.

Patient Funded Foundations

It is not uncommon for many patients with rare diseases or their families to set up support groups, particularly with the ready availability of social networking. In some cases, the only research foundations focused on particularly rare diseases have been initiated by patients and families affected by those diseases. There are over 7,000 rare genetic diseases impacting 8-10% of the US population or about 25 million patients. When such a disease afflicts a high profile or financially successful individual, or their family member, that particular disease can receive disproportionate attention and support.

Patient Funded Research

In this model, the patient pays for participating in the clinical research. In terms of the research, this is similar to the Private Funded model discussed above. Less common conditions and risky proposals may be studied, unencumbered by bureaucracy and coupled with the ability to make quick decisions.

Critics argue that desperate patients can be exploited and should not pay for clinical research. Clearly, people with resources decide how to use their resources. Not allowing patients to pay for research would restrict their ability to use their own resources as they see fit.

Unlike other types of funding, patient funded research is subject to market demands. If a study is too expensive, there will be less participants, unlike the situation where the funding is provided for the patient to participate in the research. The self-funding patient will be more inclined to demand information thus providing a more thought out informed consent than in a study where free care is provided, as they want to receive their "money's worth." One can argue that free medical care may be considered an exploitative inducement to participate in research.

Patient funded studies are generally for conditions not being investigated by NIH or pharmaceutical studies and tend towards novel approaches for less prevalent medical problems.

Patient funded research has been criticized for, by its nature, it eliminates the participation of individuals who cannot afford to participate. One can make the same criticism for the other funding sources; as unless the study pays the patient for participation, including travel costs, individuals may be unable to take the required time off from work, nor have the financial and personal support structure in place to engage in a study. Since the purpose of a research study is to determine whether the clinical intervention is of benefit, and such interventions may carry some medical risk, one could argue that aligning financial cost with participation creates a higher level of patient engagement, risk benefit assessment and therefore informed consent. In addition, the ultimate benefits of basic and clinical research accrue to all individuals with a particular disease irrespective of financial wherewithal.

Does profit taint the research? One could say that all human activity creates bias, otherwise there would be no activity. Unless the research is self-funded, researchers are always paid by some funding source; otherwise they could not perform the research. Frequently, both NIH and pharmaceutical funding is proportional to the number of subjects the researcher enrolls in the study, which some may consider to be unethical. In this respect, the patient funded study differs little from other types of studies. As pointed out previously, it is in the researcher's interest to keep the patient cost at a reasonable level in order to encourage patient entry.

This paper is a discussion of actual medical studies and does not speak to the situation in which a private physician requires a patient to pay for treatment with an off-label remedy for which no protocol has been written, there is no Institutional Review Board (IRB) approval, and no data is being collected.

The patient funded study, that has a detailed protocol, has undergone IRB review, is listed with ClinicalTrials.gov (NIH), and is publishing results, whether positive or negative, is an important form of research allowing the testing of ideas that would otherwise languish due to a lack of funding.

All human endeavors require work and effort and therefore have financial costs. There is a range of how removed the patients are from those costs, depending on the research payment methodology.

In the case of publically funded clinical research, the patient may have low awareness of the cost of the clinical research as the funds are taken from the general tax base of whose allocation individuals have minimal awareness. In publicly funded research, the cost of an individual's participation is spread out over millions of people and therefore the percentage of cost that is the responsibility of an individual patient is low. This low awareness of source and percentage cost of participation removes these particular financial considerations from the informed consent process.

On the other end of the spectrum, patient funded research causes high awareness of the cost of that individual's participation and causes a high percentage of the cost to be the responsibility of the participating patient. This high awareness enters the informed consent process as an additional consideration as patients weigh the potential personal benefit of participation. This causes a pause in this process, even for the wealthiest individuals.

Pharmaceutical clinical research would fall in-between with the actual costs being deferred to a later time, but still assumed by the individual patient needing the successfully proven care depending on the health insurance methodology.

In considering the different methods of funding of clinical research, the overall benefit of properly done clinical research, from whichever funding source, should be kept in mind. All clinical research and patient care creates costs that ultimately accrue to individuals in the society. It is only a matter of how directly those costs are felt by individuals.

Suggested Reading

1. ClinicalTrials.gov. Learn about clinical studies. Accessed December 11, 2014.
2. U.S. Investment in Health Research – Research America. Accessed December 8, 2014.
3. Parke DW. Current Perspective, Innovation: Risky Business. EyeNet. December 2014:12
4. Lind SE. Fee-for-service research. N Engl J Med 1986;314:312-315.
5. Lind SE. Dilemmas in paying for clinical research: The view from the IRBs. IRB: A Review of Human Subjects Research March/April 1987;9:1-5.
6. Lind SE. Financial issues and incentives related to clinical research and innovative therapies. In Vanderpool HY, ed. The Ethics of Research Involving Human Subjects: Facing the 21st Century. Frederick, MD: University Publishing Group, 1996:185-202.
7. Best RK. Disease politics and medical research funding: Three ways advocacy shapes policy. American Sociological Review. 2012:77(5); 780-803.
8. Kuhn T. The Structure of Scientific Revolutions. Chicago: University of Chicago Press, 1962.
9. Myers ER, Alciati, MH, Ahiport, KN, Sung, NS. Similarities and differences in philanthropic and federal support for member states: An analysis of funding by nonprofits in 2006-2008. Academic Medicine. November 2012;12(1)1574-1581.
10. Evan S, Block JB. Perspective-Ethical issues regarding fee-for-service-funded research within a complementary medicine context. Journal Alternative and Complementary Med. 7:6,2001;697-702.
11. Rose Bowl opponents team up to raise awareness of a rare blood disorder. PBS NewsHour Episode December 31, 2014 http://video.pbs.org/video/2365395300/